Coping with Childhood Leukemias

A Practical and Supportive Handbook for Families, Friends and Teachers

Dr Jacob Jabin

TABLE OF CONTENTS

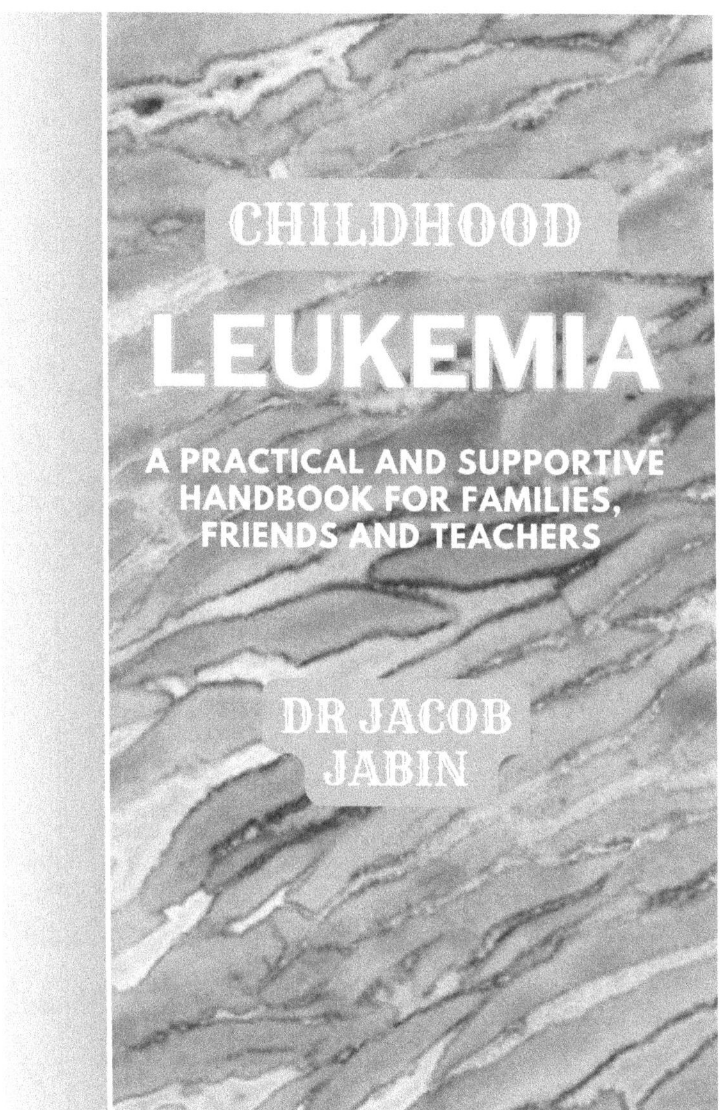
CHILDHOOD
LEUKEMIA
A PRACTICAL AND SUPPORTIVE HANDBOOK FOR FAMILIES, FRIENDS AND TEACHERS
DR JACOB JABIN

INTRODUCTION

When a kid is diagnosed with leukaemia, it is a life-changing event for the entire family. Leukaemia is a form of cancer that affects the blood cells, and it is the most frequent malignancy in children and teenagers. The treatment for leukaemia may be protracted and intense, comprising chemotherapy, radiation, and occasionally bone marrow or stem cell transplants. The therapy might induce physical and mental adverse effects, such as hair loss, nausea, exhaustion, discomfort, anxiety, and despair. The kid may have to spend a lot of time in the hospital, miss school and activities, and struggle with changes in their look and self-image. The family may have to cope with financial and practical obstacles, such as medical expenses, insurance, transportation, and daycare. The friends and instructors of the kid may also have questions and concerns about how to help the youngster and the family.

This book is meant to help you deal with the difficulties and changes that childhood leukaemia presents. It gives information and guidance on issues such as:

- The causes and kinds of paediatric leukaemia, and how it is diagnosed and staged.

- The treatment alternatives and their advantages and dangers, and how to control the side effects and consequences.

- The emotional and social effect of leukaemia on the kid and the family, and how to cope with emotions of fear, anger, guilt, and despair.

- The methods to communicate with the medical team, the family, the friends, and the teachers, and how to advocate for the child's needs and rights.

- The resources and support available for the kid and the family, such as counselling, support groups, financial aid, and educational programs.

- The long-term prognosis and follow-up care for the kid, and how to avoid and identify late consequences of therapy, such as infections, development issues, learning challenges, and secondary malignancies.

This book is presented in a straightforward and caring style, with drawings and examples to help you comprehend the medical jargon and ideas. It also offers tales and recommendations from other children and families who have gone through similar situations. It is meant for parents and caregivers of children with leukaemia, as well as their friends and instructors who wish to learn more and provide support.

We hope that this book will help you and your child fight leukaemia with bravery and optimism. Remember that you are not alone, and that there are many people who care about you and want to assist you.

CHAPTER 1

Who gets leukaemia

Leukaemia is a form of cancer that affects the blood cells, generally the white blood cells. There are numerous forms of leukaemia, and some are more frequent in specific age groups or cultures. Here is an overview of some facts regarding leukaemia:

1- Leukaemia may be characterised by how rapidly it advances (*acute or chronic*) and by the kind of blood cell affected (*myeloid or lymphoid*).

2- Acute leukaemia develops fast and demands prompt treatment. Chronic leukaemia develops slowly and may not show symptoms for years.

3- Myeloid leukaemia affects the myeloid cells, which ordinarily grow into red blood cells, platelets, and certain kinds of white blood cells. Lymphoid leukaemia affects the lymphoid cells, which usually grow into white blood cells that fight infection.

4-The most frequent kind of leukaemia in children, teenagers, and young adults up to age 39 is acute lymphoid leukaemia (ALL). The most prevalent kind of leukaemia in persons over 65 is chronic lymphoid leukaemia (CLL).

5- The most frequent kind of acute leukaemia in adults is acute myeloid leukaemia (AML). It is also more frequent in elderly persons, but may occur in youngsters as well.

6- Chronic myeloid leukaemia (CML) is more frequent in older persons, but may afflict adults of any age. It seldom happens in children.

7- Leukaemia is more frequent in elderly persons, with incidence rates climbing dramatically from roughly 55 years.

8- Leukaemia is also more prevalent in men than in females, and in whites than in other races.

9- Some risk factors for leukaemia include exposure to radiation, chemicals, or certain viruses, having a family history of leukaemia, or having certain genetic diseases, such as Down syndrome.

Leukaemia is a kind of blood cancer that impairs the development and function of white blood cells, which help fight infections.The signs and symptoms of leukaemia vary based on the kind and stage of the illness, however some frequent ones include:

1- Fatigue and weakness
2- Unexplained weight loss
3- Fever or chills
4- Frequent or severe infections
5- Swollen lymph nodes, spleen or liver
6- Easy bleeding or bruising
7- Recurrent nosebleeds
8- Tiny red patches on the skin (*petechiae*)
9- Excessive perspiration, particularly at night
10- Bone pain or tenderness
11- bone or joint pain, swelling of the belly, lack of appetite, weight loss, enlarged lymph nodes, fever, recurrent infections, and headaches.

Understanding Childhood Leukaemia

Childhood leukaemia is a kind of cancer that begins in the blood-forming cells of the bone marrow. It is the most frequent malignancy in children and teenagers, accounting for roughly 1 out of 3 cancers. There are many forms of juvenile leukaemia, depending on whether they are acute (*rapid growing*) or chronic (*slower developing*), and whether they originate in lymphoid cells or myeloid cells. The primary kinds of childhood leukaemia are:

Acute lymphoblastic leukaemia

Acute lymphoblastic leukaemia (ALL) is a kind of cancer that affects the white blood cells, which are part of the immune system. It is the most frequent kind of cancer in children, particularly between the ages of two and five. ALL may produce many symptoms, such as fever, bruising, bleeding, infections, bone pain, and swollen lymph nodes, liver, and spleen. ALL may also spread to other organs, including the brain and spinal cord.

The specific origin of ALL is not known, however several factors may raise the risk, such as genetic problems, exposure to radiation or chemicals, and aberrant immunological response to infections. To diagnose ALL, physicians need to undertake blood tests and bone marrow biopsy to screen for the presence of aberrant lymphocytes, termed blast cells. They may also undertake additional tests, such as ultrasonography, flow cytometry, and genetic studies, to detect the subtype and features of the leukaemia cells.

The major treatment for ALL is chemotherapy, which is the use of medications to destroy the cancer cells. Chemotherapy is administered in multiple stages, including as induction, consolidation, maintenance, and occasionally re-induction, depending on the response and risk of recurrence. Some children may also require radiation, which is the use of high-energy rays to eradicate the cancer cells, particularly if the leukaemia has progressed to the brain or spinal cord. Another alternative is stem cell transplant, which is the replacement of the bone marrow with healthy stem cells from a donor, generally reserved for high-risk or relapsed patients.

The prognosis of ALL relies on numerous variables, such as the age, subtype, and genetic characteristics of the leukaemia, the response to therapy, and the existence of comorbidities. The survival rate of ALL has improved dramatically over the years, mainly to breakthroughs in diagnosis and therapy. More than 90% of children with ALL reach remission, and nearly 80% of them are cured. However, therapy may also produce short-term and long-term adverse effects, such as infections, bleeding, nausea, hair loss, infertility, growth issues, and secondary malignancies. Therefore, children with ALL require frequent follow-up and supportive treatment to assess their health and quality of life.

Acute myeloid leukaemia

Acute myeloid leukaemia (AML) is a kind of cancer that affects the myeloid cells, which are a type of white blood cell that help fight infections. AML is the second most frequent kind of leukaemia in children, behind acute lymphoblastic leukaemia (ALL). AML arises when the myeloid cells expand and divide abnormally, pushing out the normal blood cells in the bone marrow and the circulation.

The signs and symptoms of AML in children may include:

- Fever, infections, and bleeding or bruising easily

- Pale skin, weakness, and weariness
- Bone or joint discomfort and swelling
- Enlarged lymph nodes, liver, or spleen
- Headaches, vomiting, or seizures - Difficulty breathing or chest discomfort

To diagnose AML in children, clinicians need to undertake blood tests and bone marrow testing to screen for the presence and kind of aberrant myeloid cells. They may also undertake additional tests, such as genetic testing, imaging tests, or lumbar puncture, to establish the subtype and features of the leukaemia cells and to detect whether the leukaemia has spread to other organs, such as the brain or spinal cord.

The therapy for AML in children relies on numerous aspects, such as the subtype, risk category, and response to treatment. The major treatment is chemotherapy, which is the use of medications to destroy the cancer cells. Chemotherapy is administered in multiple stages, including as induction, consolidation, and maintenance, depending on the purpose and result of each phase. Some children may additionally require extra therapies, such as:

1- Stem cell transplant, which is the replacement of the bone marrow with healthy stem cells from a donor, mainly reserved for high-risk or relapsed patients.

2- Radiotherapy, which is the use of high-energy radiation to eliminate cancer cells, particularly if the leukaemia has gone to the brain or spinal cord.

3- Targeted treatment, which involves the use of medications that target particular properties of the leukaemia cells, such as mutations or receptors.

4- Immunotherapy, which is the use of medications that activate the immune system to combat the cancer cells, such as antibodies or vaccines

The prognosis of AML in children relies on numerous variables, such as the age, subtype, and genetic aspects of the leukaemia, the response to therapy, and the occurrence of comorbidities. The survival rate of AML in children has improved dramatically over the years, mainly due to breakthroughs in diagnosis and therapy. roughly 70% of children with AML reach remission, and roughly 60% of them are cured. However, therapy may also produce short-term and long-term adverse effects, such as infections, bleeding, nausea, hair loss, infertility, growth issues, and secondary malignancies. Therefore, children with AML require frequent follow-up and supportive care to assess their health and quality of life.

Juvenile myelomonocytic leukaemia

JMML is an uncommon and deadly kind of blood cancer that affects young children, generally under 4 years old. It happens when too many immature white blood cells termed monocytes and myelocytes are generated in the bone marrow and push out the regular blood cells. JMML may potentially extend to other organs such as the skin, lungs, liver, or intestines.

The symptoms of JMML differ from kid to child, however some frequent ones are:

- Fever for no known cause
- Infections, such as bronchitis or tonsillitis
- Feeling very tired
- Easy bruising or bleeding of the skin, nose, and mouth
- Red skin rash or tiny, red pinpoint dots on the skin
- Painless swelling of the lymph nodes in the neck, underarm, stomach, or groyne
- Pain or a feeling of fullness below the ribs
- Dry cough
- Trouble gaining weight
- Poor appetite
- Failure to thrive
- Feeling irritable

- Enlarged spleen or liver
- Anaemia

The specific aetiology of JMML is not understood, however it is connected to changes in genes that affect the formation and development of blood cells. Some children with a hereditary disease called neurofibromatosis type 1 (NF1) have an increased chance of developing JMML.

The diagnosis of JMML is based on the findings of blood testing, bone marrow tests, and genetic tests. The prognosis of JMML relies on various variables, such as the age of the child, the genetic alterations implicated, and the response to therapy.

The only therapy that gives promise of a long-term cure for JMML is allogeneic stem cell transplantation, which utilises healthy stem cells from a donor to replace the aberrant blood cells in the child's bone marrow. This treatment should be done as soon as feasible following diagnosis, since it has better results in younger children. However, stem cell transplantation is a difficult and hazardous process that needs a good donor and specialised care. Other therapies, like chemotherapy and immunotherapy, may be used to reduce the symptoms and prepare the kid for transplantation.

The survival statistics for JMML vary depending on the source of information, but usually, roughly 50% of children with JMML are treated after stem cell transplantation. However, some children may relapse or have difficulties following transplantation.

What is Blast

A blast is an immature blood cell that generally remains in the bone marrow until it grows. In paediatric leukaemia, the bone marrow creates too many blasts that do not function correctly and push out the healthy blood cells. There are many forms of blasts, such as lymphoid blasts or myeloid blasts, depending on the type of leukaemia. Blasts may also travel to other regions of the body, such as the central nervous system, producing difficulties.

There are two basic kinds of blast cells that may develop leukaemia in children: **lymphoid blasts** and **myeloid blasts.** These cells are immature types of white blood cells that ordinarily evolve into lymphocytes and myelocytes, respectively. Lymphocytes and myelocytes are elements of the immune system and help fight infections.

Lymphoid blasts produce acute lymphoblastic leukaemia (ALL), which is the most frequent form of paediatric leukaemia. It accounts for around 75% of all instances[1]. Myeloid blasts produce acute myeloid leukaemia (AML), which is the second most frequent kind of juvenile leukaemia. It accounts for around 20% of all cases.

The specific reasons of blast cell overproduction are not fully known, however they are likely connected to genetic mutations or alterations in the DNA of the cells. Some of these mutations may be inherited from parents, while others may emerge randomly during the child's growth or exposure to environmental influences.

The biology and genetics of paediatric leukaemia

The biology and genetics of paediatric leukaemia are complicated and not entirely understood. Some variables that may contribute to the development of paediatric leukaemia are:

- Genetic mutations: These are alterations in the DNA of the blood cells that cause them to develop and divide abnormally. Some mutations may be inherited from the parents, while others may emerge spontaneously or due to environmental exposures. Some examples of genetic mutations that are related with paediatric leukaemia include:

- Translocations: These are rearrangements of portions of chromosomes (the structures that hold the genes). For example, the Philadelphia chromosome is a translocation between chromosomes 9 and 22 that is observed in most instances of CML and certain cases of ALL.

- Deletions: These are losses of sections of chromosomes. For example, the 11q23 deletion is a loss of part of chromosome 11 that is detected in certain instances of AML and ALL.

- Duplications: These are gains of sections of chromosomes. For example, trisomy 21 is a duplication of chromosome 21 that is present in certain instances of AML and ALL, notably in children with Down syndrome.

- Point mutations: These are alterations in single nucleotides (the building units of DNA). For example, the FLT3 mutation is an alteration in a gene that is identified in certain instances of AML and ALL.

- **Inherited syndromes:** These are disorders that are handed down from the parents and enhance the likelihood of developing childhood leukaemia.

Some examples of hereditary disorders that are related with childhood leukaemia include:

- **Down syndrome:** This is a disorder that is caused by having an extra copy of chromosome 21. It raises the chance of acquiring AML and ALL, particularly after the age of 5.

- **Fanconi anaemia:** This is a disorder that is caused by mutations in genes that are involved in DNA repair. It raises the chance of acquiring AML and other malignancies.

- **Li-Fraumeni syndrome:** This is a disorder that is caused by mutations in the TP53 gene, which is a tumour suppressor gene. It raises the chance of getting AML, ALL, and other malignancies.

- **Neurofibromatosis type 1:** This is a disorder that is caused by mutations in the NF1 gene, which is a tumour suppressor gene. It raises the chance of acquiring JMML and other malignancies.

- **Environmental variables:** These are factors that are connected to the surroundings or lifestyle of the kid or the parents that may raise the chance of developing childhood leukaemia. Some examples of environmental variables that are connected with childhood leukaemia include:

- **Ionising radiation:** This is a form of radiation that may harm the DNA of the cells. It may arise from sources such as x-rays, nuclear mishaps, or atomic weapons. It raises the likelihood of developing AML, ALL, and CML.
- **Chemical exposures:** These are chemicals that might harm the DNA of the cells or interfere with their normal function. They may arise from sources such as insecticides, solvents, or tobacco smoke. They may raise the likelihood of developing AML, ALL, or CML.
- **Infections:** These are illnesses that are caused by viruses, bacteria, or other microorganisms that might harm the immune system or the blood cells. They may occur from origins such as chickenpox, hepatitis B, or human immunodeficiency virus (HIV). They may raise or reduce the chance of developing AML, ALL, or CML, depending on the nature and time of the infection.

Statistics and numbers concerning the epidemiology and risk factors of paediatric leukaemia

The epidemiology and risk factors of juvenile leukaemia involve the study of how frequently it happens, where it occurs, and what impacts its incidence. Some statistics and numbers concerning the epidemiology and risk factors of paediatric leukaemia are:

1- Childhood leukaemia is more prevalent in males than in girls, and in white children than in black children.

2- Childhood leukaemia is more frequent in affluent nations than in undeveloped countries.

3- juvenile leukaemia accounts for around 25% of all juvenile malignancies and 3% of all cancers in the United States.

4- The incidence (new cases) of juvenile leukaemia in the United States is around 4.8 per 100,000 children per year.

5-The mortality (deaths) of juvenile leukaemia in the United States is around 0.6 per 100,000 children per year.

6- The survival rate (probability of surviving at least 5 years following diagnosis) of juvenile leukaemia in the United States is around 86%.

7- The risk factors for juvenile leukaemia are not fully defined, although some plausible causes include genetic mutations, hereditary disorders, environmental factors, and infections.

CHAPTER 2

Techniques to detect childhood leukaemia

Childhood leukaemia is a kind of blood cancer that affects the development and function of white blood cells. It is the most frequent malignancy in children, accounting for around 30% of all paediatric cancers. The signs and symptoms of paediatric leukaemia may include fever, exhaustion, bruises, bleeding, infections, bone or joint pain, swollen lymph nodes, enlarged spleen or liver, and weight loss.

To diagnose paediatric leukaemia, physicians normally run a battery of tests on blood and bone marrow samples, as well as other tests to evaluate the degree of the illness and its subtype. Some of the frequent tests are:

1- Blood tests: A complete blood count (CBC) evaluates the quantity and type of blood cells in a sample. A blood smear studies the form and size of blood cells under a microscope. Children with leukaemia generally have too many immature white blood cells (called blasts) and not enough red blood cells or platelets.

2- Bone marrow tests: A bone marrow aspiration or biopsy extracts a tiny quantity of bone marrow fluid or tissue from the hip bone or other bones. The sample is next evaluated for the existence and proportion of leukaemia cells, as well as their genetic and molecular properties.

3- Genetic testing: These tests check for particular abnormalities or mutations in the DNA of leukaemia cells, such as translocations, deletions, or duplications. These alterations may assist identify the subtype of leukaemia and its prognosis, as well as advise the choice of therapy.

4- Minimal residual disease (MRD) test: This test assesses the quantity of leukaemia cells that remain in the blood or bone marrow following therapy. It may assist in measuring the response to therapy and the likelihood of recurrence.

5- Lumbar puncture: Also known as a spinal tap, this test involves inserting a needle into the lower back and collecting some cerebrospinal fluid (CSF), which surrounds the brain and spinal cord. The CSF is then tested for leukaemia cells or evidence of infection. This test may assist establish whether the leukaemia has progressed to the central nervous system (CNS).

6- Imaging tests: These tests employ x-rays, sound waves, magnetic fields, or radioactive chemicals to generate images of the interior of the body. They may assist identify the size and location of organs, lymph nodes, or malignancies. Some of the typical imaging tests for children with leukaemia include chest x-ray, ultrasound, computed tomography (CT) scan, magnetic resonance imaging (MRI) scan, and positron emission tomography (PET) scan.

The present research and discoveries in the area of children's leukaemia

The present research and discoveries in the area of children's leukaemia are focused at increasing the knowledge, diagnosis, treatment, and prevention of the illness. Some examples of current research and achievements in the area of children leukaemia are:

1- Molecular profiling: This is the investigation of the genetic and molecular properties of the leukaemia cells, such as the mutations, translocations, deletions, duplications, and point mutations. This may assist to categorise the leukaemia into subgroups, forecast the prognosis, and guide the treatment.

2- Immunotherapy: This is the use of the immune system or its components to attack leukaemia cells. This may involve the use of monoclonal antibodies, chimeric antigen receptor (CAR) T cells, or vaccines.

3- Targeted therapy: This is the use of medications that precisely target the aberrant proteins or pathways that are involved in the development and survival of the leukaemia cells. This may involve the use of tyrosine kinase inhibitors, BCL-2 inhibitors, or FLT3 inhibitors.

4-Stem cell transplantation: This is the operation of replacing the bone marrow of the kid with healthy stem cells from a donor or from the child's own blood or umbilical cord blood. This may assist to restore the normal blood production and destroy the leukaemia cells.

5- Clinical trials: These are studies that evaluate novel medications, combinations of treatments, or techniques of therapy in children with leukaemia. They can assist to find out whether the new therapies are safe and effective.

The challenges and constraints in the realm of childhood leukaemia are the hurdles or problems that inhibit the development or improvement of the illness. Some examples of obstacles and constraints in the realm of childhood leukaemia are:

1-Side effects: These are the undesirable or dangerous results of the therapy, such as infections, bleeding, nausea, vomiting, hair loss, or organ damage. They may impact the quality of life and the long-term health of the child.

2- Resistance: This is the capacity of the leukaemia cells to survive or grow despite the therapy, such as by generating new mutations or activating alternate pathways. It may impair the efficacy and the length of the treatment.

3- Relapse: This is the return of the leukaemia after a time of remission (no signs or symptoms of the illness). It may arise in the bone marrow or in other regions of the body, such as the brain, the spinal cord, or the testicles. It may be tougher to cure and have a poorer prognosis than the original leukaemia.

4- Disparities: These are the disparities or inequalities in the incidence, outcome, or access to care of the illness, such as by race, ethnicity, gender, age, location, or socioeconomic position. They may alter the risk, diagnosis, treatment, and survival of the child.

5- Prevention: This is the activity or measure that may minimise the possibility of acquiring the illness, such as by avoiding or limiting the exposure to the risk factors, or by boosting the protective factors. It is not well established for childhood leukaemia, since most of the risk variables are either changeable or not fully understood.

Central venous catheters

CVCs are tubes that are put into a major vein in the arm, neck, chest or groyne and into the central blood circulation. They are also known as central venous access devices (CVADs). CVCs are used for obtaining blood samples, delivering fluids, blood, chemotherapy and other medications without the need for frequent needle pricks.

CVCs are especially important for children with leukaemia, since they require regular blood tests and medications that may be administered via the CVC. CVCs may lessen the discomfort and stress of getting injections and blood draws, and can also lower the risk of infection and bleeding from the injection sites. CVCs may be either temporary or permanent, depending on the kind and length of therapy. Some popular kinds of CVCs are:

1- a Hickman line: This is a long, thin tube that is put into a vein in the chest and comes out through the skin on the chest or belly. It features one or more apertures (lumens) at the end that may be capped or attached to a drip or syringe.

2- PICC line (peripherally implanted central catheter line): This is commonly placed into a big vein in the arm. It has the same purpose as a Hickman line, but it is shorter and simpler to put and remove.

3- implanted port: This is a tiny device that is put under the skin on the chest or belly. It has a chamber (port) that links to a vein by a thin tube (catheter). A specific needle is used to access the port and give medications or fluids.

CVCs need to be cared after carefully to avoid problems like :
- infection,
- obstruction,
- leaking,
- dislodgement.

The CVC site should be maintained clean and dry, and the dressing should be changed routinely. The CVC should be flushed with saline or heparin solution to maintain it clean and avoid blood clots. Any indications of redness, swelling, discomfort, fever, or pus around the CVC site should be reported to the doctor promptly.

CVCs may potentially raise the risk of venous thromboembolism (VTE), which is the production of blood clots in the veins. VTE may create major complications such as pulmonary embolism (PE), which is when a blood clot goes to the lungs and stops the blood flow. VTE may be avoided and treated using anticoagulant medications, such as warfarin or low molecular weight heparin (LMWH).
- CVCs are normally removed after the therapy is done or no longer required. The removal technique is normally done under local anesthesia and is rapid and painless. The CVC site may be uncomfortable for a few days and may leave a minor scar.

Catheters may offer certain advantages, such as minimising the discomfort and stress of having injections and blood draws, lowering the risk of infection and bleeding from the injection sites, and avoiding urine accumulation and kidney damage.
 However, catheters may also have certain downsides, such as raising the risk of infection, obstruction, leakage, or dislodgement of the catheter, requiring meticulous maintenance and cleanliness, and causing pain, irritation, or humiliation.

Some children with leukaemia may opt not to use a catheter for personal, medical, or practical reasons. For example, some children may choose to employ different techniques of bladder management, such as intermittent catheterization, bladder training, medication, or surgery. Some children may have allergies or sensitivities to the catheter materials, or develop problems from the catheter, such as blood clots or allergic reactions. Some children may find the catheter difficult, pricey, or unsuited for their lifestyle or tastes.

- Choosing not to use a catheter is a personal choice that should be taken in conjunction with the doctor and based on the child's health, requirements, and objectives. The doctor may give information and advice on the advantages and drawbacks of using or not utilising a catheter, and the various alternatives and their risks and benefits. - If a kid prefers not to use a catheter, they should follow the doctor's advice on how to maintain their bladder function, check their pee flow and quality, and avoid or treat any issues that may emerge. They should also seek medical assistance if they have any indications of infection, bleeding, discomfort, or problems urinating.

Coping with Diagnosis and Treatment

When a kid is diagnosed with a severe disease, it can be a very tough and stressful period for the entire family. The youngster may feel fear, rage, grief, uncertainty, or guilt. The parents may feel overwhelmed, scared, powerless, or guilty. The siblings may feel ignored, envious, or resentful. The family may also confront practical hurdles such as financial difficulties, transportation constraints, or childcare arrangements.

It is crucial to manage these emotions and problems in a healthy and productive manner. Here are some recommendations on how to achieve that:

1- Communicate with the child: Depending on the child's age and maturity level, describe the diagnosis and therapy in a straightforward and honest manner. Use basic and precise terms that the youngster can comprehend. Avoid offering false reassurances or suppressing facts. Encourage the child to ask inquiries and share their emotions. Listen to the children and validate their feelings. Provide comfort and support. Involve the children in decision-making as much as possible. Help the youngster retain a feeling of normality and regularity by maintaining their schooling, hobbies, and social activities as much as possible.

2- Communicate with the medical team: Establish a good connection with the physicians, nurses, and other health care workers who are treating the kid. Ask questions and seek clarity on the diagnosis, prognosis, treatment choices, side effects, complications, and long-term impacts. Share any concerns or preferences you have concerning the child's care. Follow the treatment plan and instructions attentively. Keep a record of the child's medical history, test results, prescriptions, and appointments. Seek a second opinion if you are unclear or unsatisfied with the therapy.

3- Communicate with other family members and friends: Share the diagnostic and treatment information with the child's siblings, grandparents, relatives, and close friends. Explain how the disease and treatment may impact the kid and the family. Ask for their aid and support. Be attentive to their emotions and responses.

Keep them informed on the child's development and condition. Acknowledge and appreciate their work and contributions. Spend quality time with them and show them that you care.

4- Manage the side effects, complications, and long-term consequences of therapy: Learn about the probable side effects, complications, and long-term impacts of the treatment. Be prepared for them and know how to avoid, identify, and treat them. Follow the advice and suggestions of the medical team. Seek medical treatment if the kid suffers any severe or unexpected symptoms. Monitor the child's physical and mental health frequently. Help the youngster manage with discomfort, nausea, exhaustion, hair loss, infections, or other difficulties. Provide proper diet, water, relaxation, and cleanliness. Help the youngster adapt to any changes in their look, talents, or lifestyle.

5- Seek professional assistance: If the kid or the family is dealing with the emotional, psychological, or social elements of coping with the diagnosis and treatment, seek professional support from a counsellor, therapist, psychologist, psychiatrist, or social worker. They may give counselling, therapy, medicine, or other treatments to assist the kid and the family with stress, anxiety, sadness, grief, trauma, or other challenges. They may also make references to other resources or services that may be beneficial, such as support groups, financial aid, legal counsel, or educational assistance.

6- Take care of yourself: As a parent or caregiver, it is crucial to take care of your own physical, mental, and emotional well-being. Do not disregard your own health, needs, or hobbies. Eat healthy, exercise, sleep, and relax. Find healthy methods to deal with stress, such as meditation, yoga, music, painting, or hobbies. Seek help from your spouse, partner, family, friends, or other caregivers. Join a support group or online community of parents or caregivers who are going through similar situations. Seek aid from others when you need it. Do not feel guilty or embarrassed to seek assistance. Remember that you are not alone and that you are trying your best.

CHAPTER 3

Chemotherapy and other drugs

Chemotherapy is the principal treatment for most paediatric leukaemias. It is the use of anti-cancer medications that destroy or inhibit the proliferation of leukaemia cells. Chemotherapy may be delivered in several methods, such as via a vein (IV), in a muscle, in the fluid surrounding the brain and spinal cord (CSF), or by mouth. Chemotherapy is frequently administered in cycles, with periods of treatment followed by periods of relaxation. The medications, dosages, and regimens vary based on the kind and stage of leukaemia.

Some of the common chemotherapeutic medicines used for juvenile leukaemia are:

1- Vincristine: This medicine interferes with the division of leukaemia cells and causes them to die. It is administered as an IV injection, generally once a week. It may produce negative effects such as hair loss, nerve damage, constipation, and mouth sores.

2- L-asparaginase: This medicine breaks down a protein called asparagine, which leukaemia cells require to live. It is administered as an IV injection or a shot in a muscle, generally two or three times a week. It may produce negative effects including allergic reactions, pancreatitis, blood clotting issues, and liver damage.

3- Steroids: These medications are hormones that help decrease inflammation and slow down the proliferation of leukaemia cells. They may be administered by mouth, as an IV injection, or as a shot in a muscle. They are normally administered for a few weeks at a time. They may produce negative effects including increased hunger, weight gain, mood changes, elevated blood pressure, and higher risk of infections.

4- Anthracyclines: These medications are antibiotics that damage the DNA of leukaemia cells and prevent them from dividing. They are administered as an IV injection, generally once every few weeks. They may induce negative effects including heart damage, nausea, vomiting, and low blood cell counts.

5- Cytarabine: This medicine is a synthetic version of a DNA building block that leukaemia cells require to proliferate. It is administered as an IV injection, generally for multiple days in a succession. It might produce adverse effects such as fever, infection, bleeding, and eye discomfort.

6- Methotrexate: This medicine prevents the generation of a vitamin that leukaemia cells require to develop. It is administered by mouth, as an IV injection, or as an injection into the CSF. It may produce negative effects such as renal damage, mouth sores, nausea, vomiting, and skin rashes.

 7- Thioguanine: These medications are also synthetic versions of DNA building components that leukaemia cells require to proliferate. They are administered by mouth, generally once a day. They may induce adverse effects including liver damage, nausea, vomiting, and low blood cell counts.

Other drugs that may be used for childhood leukaemia include:

1- Targeted therapy: These medications target particular properties of leukaemia cells, such as proteins or genes, that make them distinct from normal cells. They may be administered by mouth or as an IV injection. They may produce negative effects including skin issues, diarrhoea, high blood pressure, and bleeding.

2- Immunotherapy: These medications employ the body's immune system to combat leukaemia cells. They may be administered by mouth, as an IV injection, or as a shot under the skin. They may produce adverse effects such as fever, chills, tiredness, and allergic reactions.

3- Stem cell transplant: This is a technique that replaces the child's bone marrow, which is the source of blood cells, with healthy bone marrow from a donor. This may be done after heavy doses of chemotherapy or radiation treatment that damage the child's own bone marrow. It may produce negative effects including infection, graft-versus-host disease, and organ damage.

Chemotherapy and other drugs are beneficial in treating juvenile leukaemia, but they may also produce short-term and long-term negative effects. Some of the probable long-term impacts are:

- Growth difficulties
- Learning challenges
- Infertility - Secondary cancers
- Heart problems
- Lung issues
- Bone issues

Therefore, children with leukaemia require continuous follow-up treatment and monitoring to assess their health and growth.

Prophylactic antibiotics

Prophylactic antibiotics are medications that are used to prevent bacterial infections in patients who have a compromised immune system, such as children with leukaemia. Leukaemia is a form of cancer that affects the blood cells, and it may leave the body more susceptible to infections by diminishing the quantity of white blood cells that fight pathogens. Prophylactic antibiotics may minimise the risk of major complications and mortality from infections in children with leukaemia, particularly during the first month of treatment when the chemotherapy is most vigorous.

However, preventive antibiotics are not indicated for all children with leukaemia, since they may have certain downsides, such as side effects, drug resistance, and fungal infections. The choice to take preventive antibiotics relies on various criteria, such as the kind and stage of leukaemia, the type and length of chemotherapy, the patient's age and general health, and the local infection rates and antibiotic policy. varied clinical guidelines and research may have varied recommendations for preventive antibiotics in children with leukaemia.

According to a new guideline for antibacterial prophylaxis administration in paediatric cancer and hematopoietic stem cell transplantation, the following recommendations are provided for children with leukaemia:

- A weak recommendation for systemic antibacterial prophylaxis for children undergoing intense treatment for acute myeloid leukaemia and relapsed acute lymphoblastic leukaemia (ALL).

- A weak recommendation against the usual use of systemic antibacterial prophylaxis for children receiving induction chemotherapy for ALL, autologous HSCT and allogeneic HSCT.

- A strong recommendation against the regular use of systemic antibacterial prophylaxis for children whose medication is not predicted to result in sustained severe neutropenia.

- If administered, prophylaxis with levofloxacin is advised during severe neutropenia.

According to research by the Dana-Farber malignancy Institute (DFCI) ALL Consortium, prophylactic antibiotics greatly lowered the incidence of catastrophic bacterial infections in children during the crucial first month of therapy for ALL, the most prevalent paediatric malignancy. The research introduced universal antibiotic prophylaxis to its 11-001 treatment regimen for paediatric ALL, and found that prophylactic antibiotic therapy decreased the incidence of infection by around 60 percent compared to historic controls.

According to an article on how to treat paediatric acute myeloid leukaemia, the most consistent conclusion across multiple trials is that resistance to the antibiotic used for prophylaxis is raised, but there is no solid evidence of cross-resistance to other antibiotics. The report also indicates that antibiotic prophylaxis with levofloxacin is highly advised for all patients treated on the COG AAML1831 study.

Colony stimulating factors

CSFs are chemicals that encourage the generation and maturation of blood cells in the bone marrow. They are naturally created by the body, but they may also be administered as medications to individuals who have low blood counts owing to illnesses such as leukaemia or treatments like chemotherapy. CSFs include granulocyte colony-stimulating factor (G-CSF), granulocyte-macrophage colony-stimulating factor (GM-CSF), and erythropoietin (EPO).

CSFs are occasionally used for children with leukaemia to prevent or cure issues caused by low blood counts, such as febrile neutropenia (*a condition when the patient has a fever and a very low number of neutrophils, a kind of white blood cell that fights infections*). CSFs may also help lower the length and severity of chemotherapy-induced myelosuppression (*a condition where the bone marrow is injured by the medications and cannot create enough blood cells*).

However, CSFs are not advised for all children with leukaemia, since they may contain certain downsides, such as side effects, increased risk of recurrence, and interference with therapy effectiveness. The choice to utilise CSFs relies on various considerations, including the kind and stage of leukaemia, the type and length of chemotherapy, the patient's age and general health, and the local infection rates and antibiotic policy. varied clinical guidelines and research may have varied recommendations for CSFs in children with leukaemia.

According to a Cochrane review, there is inadequate data to support or contradict the use of CSFs for prevention of febrile neutropenia in children with ALL. The analysis indicated that CSFs may lower the incidence of febrile neutropenia episodes, but they may also raise the risk of bone discomfort and allergic responses. The study also showed no obvious impact of

CSFs on overall mortality, recurrence, hospitalisation, or treatment delays.

According to a guidance from Alex's Lemonade Stand Foundation, CSFs are not routinely utilised for children with ALL, unless they experience chronic and substantially low blood counts. They are occasionally used for children with AML or for individuals who receive stem cell transplants. The guidance adds that CSFs may lower the severity and duration of low white blood counts, decreasing the likelihood of infection, but they can also induce adverse effects such as bone pain, fever, and rash.

According to a PDQ review from the National Cancer Institute, CSF3R is the gene encoding the G-CSF receptor, and activating mutations in CSF3R are reported in 2% to 3% of juvenile AML cases. These mutations lead to increased signalling via the G-CSF receptor, and they are typically detected in AML with either CEBPA mutations or with core binding factor (CBF) abnormalities. The summary also notes that antimicrobial prophylaxis with levofloxacin is highly advised for all patients treated on the COG AAML1831 trial, which is a phase III investigation of conventional chemotherapy with or without bortezomib in newly diagnosed AML.

Anti Nausea medicines used during chemotherapy

Chemotherapy is a treatment that employs medications to destroy cancer cells, but it may also induce nausea and vomiting in certain individuals. Nausea and vomiting may influence the quality of life, nutrition, and hydration of children with leukaemia, and may interfere with their ability to take the full amount of chemotherapy.

To prevent or lessen nausea and vomiting, physicians may administer anti-nausea medications, also known as antiemetics, before, during, or after chemotherapy. These medications act by inhibiting the impulses that produce nausea and vomiting in the brain or stomach.

There are several kinds of anti-nausea medications, and they may be taken in many methods, such as by mouth, injection, infusion, or patch. Some of the common anti-nausea medicines used for childhood leukaemia are:

- **Aprepitant (Emend®):** This medicine inhibits a chemical called substance P, which is implicated in nausea and vomiting. It is commonly administered as a capsule by mouth or an infusion in a vein before chemotherapy. It may interfere with other medicines, so the pharmacist should know about all the drugs the kid takes.

- Diphenhydramine (Benadryl®): This medicine belongs to a category of drugs called antihistamines, which inhibit the effects of histamine, a chemical that may trigger nausea and vomiting. It is commonly administered as a liquid, tablet, or capsule by mouth, or an injection in a vein or muscle every 6 to 8 hours. It may produce sleepiness, dizziness, dry mouth, or excitability in young children.

- Granisetron (Granisol®, Kytril®, Sancuso®): This medicine belongs to a category of pharmaceuticals called serotonin antagonists, which inhibit the effects of serotonin, a neurotransmitter that may produce nausea and vomiting. It is commonly administered as a tablet by mouth, an injection in a vein, or a patch on the skin 30 minutes before chemotherapy. It may induce headaches, diarrhoea, constipation, high blood pressure, lethargy, fever, allergic response, or irregular heart rhythms.

- Lorazepam (Ativan®): This medicine belongs to a category of pharmaceuticals called benzodiazepines, which have sedative, anti-anxiety, and anti-nausea actions. It is commonly administered as a tablet or liquid by mouth, a pill dissolved under the tongue, or an injection in a vein, muscle, or beneath the skin. It may produce sleepiness, dizziness, decreased coordination, or memory issues.

- **Ondansetron (Zofran®):** This medicine belongs to the same category of pharmaceuticals as granisetron, and functions in a similar fashion. It is commonly administered as a tablet or liquid by mouth, or an injection or infusion in a vein. It may induce headaches, diarrhoea, constipation, or irregular heart rhythms.

- **Prochlorperazine (Compazine®):** This medicine belongs to a category of pharmaceuticals called phenothiazines, which inhibit the effects of dopamine, a neurotransmitter that may produce nausea and vomiting. It is commonly administered as a tablet or liquid by mouth, or an injection or suppository in the rectum. It may induce drowsiness, dizziness, blurred vision, dry mouth, low blood pressure, or mobility issues.

- **Promethazine (Phenergan®):** This medicine belongs to the same category of pharmaceuticals as prochlorperazine, and functions in a similar fashion. It is commonly administered as a tablet or liquid by mouth, or an injection in a vein or muscle. It may have the same negative effects as prochlorperazine, as well as skin irritation or injury if injected into a vein.

The choice of anti-nausea medications depends on the kind and amount of chemotherapy, the child's age, weight, medical history, and preferences, and the probable adverse effects and interactions of the drugs.

The doctor may prescribe one or more anti-nausea medicines, and change the dosage and schedule as required. The kid should take the anti-nausea medications as indicated, and report any adverse effects or concerns to the doctor or nurse.

Anti-nausea medications may help make chemotherapy more comfortable for children with leukaemia, but they are not always successful or without adverse effects. Therefore, various actions may also help avoid or decrease nausea and vomiting, such as:

- Eating small, regular, bland meals and snacks
- Avoiding spicy, fatty, or strong smelling meals and beverages
- Drinking lots of fluids, particularly water, ginger ale, or clear broth
- Sucking on ice chips, popsicles, or hard sweets
- Using relaxation methods, such as deep breathing, meditation, or music
- Distracting the youngster with games, books, or toys - Seeking emotional support from family, friends, or counsellors

Nausea and vomiting are typical and unpleasant side effects of chemotherapy, although they may be controlled using anti-nausea medicines and other techniques. By avoiding or minimising nausea and vomiting, children with leukaemia may have a higher quality of life and a greater chance of finishing their treatment successfully.

Pain eased medications

Children with leukaemia may suffer pain from numerous causes, such as the illness itself, the therapies, the testing, or the side effects of the medications. Pain may influence the child's physical, emotional, and social well-being, and interfere with their everyday activities and quality of life. Therefore, pain treatment is a crucial element of the child's care.

There are various forms of pain management medicines, generally known as analgesics, that may be used for children with leukaemia. These medications act by inhibiting the impulses that produce pain in the brain or nerves. They may be administered in numerous methods, such as via mouth, injection, infusion, patch, or pump. Some of the common pain management medicines used for childhood leukaemia are:

1- Non-opioids: These medicines include acetaminophen (Tylenol®) and non-steroidal anti-inflammatory drugs (NSAIDs), such as ibuprofen (Advil®, Motrin®) and naproxen (Aleve®). They are typically beneficial for mild to moderate discomfort, such as headaches, muscular pains, or fever. They may be delivered as tablets, liquids, or suppositories. They may produce negative effects such as stomach distress, bleeding, liver damage, or kidney damage, particularly if used for a long period or in large doses.

2- Opioids: These medicines include morphine, hydromorphone (Dilaudid®), oxycodone (OxyContin®, Percocet®), fentanyl (Duragesic®, Actiq®), and methadone. They are typically beneficial for moderate to severe pain, such as bone pain, nerve pain, or pain following surgery or treatments. They may be delivered as tablets, liquids, injections, infusions, patches, or lozenges. They may produce adverse effects such as sleepiness, nausea, constipation, itching, or breathing issues. They may also induce dependency or addiction if overused or abused.

3- Adjuvants: These medications include antidepressants, anticonvulsants, steroids, and local anaesthetics. They are frequently used combined with non-opioids or opioids to increase their pain reduction benefits, or to treat particular forms of pain, such as nerve pain, inflammation, or neuropathy. They may be delivered as tablets, liquids, injections, infusions, or lotions. They may produce adverse effects such as dry mouth, dizziness, weight gain, mood changes, or skin irritation.

The choice of pain treatment medicines relies on the kind, severity, location, and duration of the pain, as well as the child's age, weight, medical history, and preferences. The doctor may prescribe one or more pain management medicines, and change the dosage and schedule as required. The kid should take the pain management medicines as indicated, and report any adverse effects or concerns to the doctor or nurse.

Pain management medicines may help lessen the pain and improve the comfort of children with leukaemia, however they are not always effective or without adverse effects. Therefore, additional methods may also assist alleviate pain, such as:

- Applying heat or cold packs to the painful area
- Massaging or massaging the painful area
- Using distraction strategies, such as games, music, or movies
- Using relaxation methods, such as deep breathing, meditation, or hypnosis
- Seeking emotional support from family, friends, or counsellors

Pain is a frequent and frustrating symptom of leukaemia, although it may be treated with pain treatment medicines and other measures. By reducing pain, children with leukaemia may have a better quality of life

and a higher chance of dealing with their treatment and
recovery.

Complementary therapy refers to therapies that are
used combined with regular medical care to aid boost
the physical and emotional well-being of patients.
Complementary medicine does not guarantee to cure
cancer, but it may help alleviate some of the symptoms
and side effects of cancer and its therapy.
Complementary therapy is separate from alternative
treatment, which is utilised instead of established
medical care and may be harmful or ineffective.

There are numerous sorts of complementary therapies
that may be effective for children with leukaemia, such
as:

1- Acupuncture: This is an ancient Chinese practice
that entails inserting tiny needles into specified spots on
the body to promote the flow of qi and alleviate pain,
illness, or worry.

2- Aromatherapy: This is the use of natural oils derived from plants to increase mood, relaxation, or sleep. The oils may be inhaled, massaged onto the skin, or added to baths or diffusers.

3- Hypnotherapy: This is a form of guided relaxation that includes suggestions to aid the patient cope with tension, discomfort, or worry. It may also aid with activities such as smoking or overeating.

4- Massage: This is the manipulation of the muscles and soft tissues of the body to enhance blood circulation, alleviate tension, and induce relaxation. Massage may also aid with pain, exhaustion, or anxiety.

5- Reflexology: This is a sort of massage that applies pressure to certain places on the feet, hands, or ears that correlate to various organs or systems in the body. Reflexology may assist with pain, nausea, or tension.

6- Yoga: This is a system of physical exercises, breathing methods, and meditation that originated in India. Yoga may aid with flexibility, strength, balance, and relaxation. Yoga may also aid with mood, sleep, or exhaustion.

The choice of complementary treatments relies on the preferences, requirements, and objectives of the patient and their family. Some factors to consider are:

- The availability, affordability, and safety of the treatment
- The evidence and research supporting the therapy
- The potential advantages and hazards of the therapy
- The probable combinations of the therapy with other treatments or drugs
- The credentials and expertise of the therapist

Before initiating any complementary treatment, it is necessary to discuss it with the child's medical team and gain their agreement. The medical staff may also give information and recommendations to recognized and trusted sources of alternative treatments. The kid should continue to follow their recommended treatment plan and report any changes or concerns to their doctor or nurse.

Complementary treatments may be a beneficial supplement to the normal treatment of childhood leukaemia, since they may assist enhance the quality of life and well-being of the child and their family. However, they are not a replacement for medical treatment and should be taken with caution and supervision.

Treatment for children leukaemia typically includes chemotherapy, which is the use of chemicals to destroy cancer cells. Sometimes, alternative therapies like radiation therapy, targeted therapy, immunotherapy, or stem cell transplant may also be employed. These therapies may be quite beneficial, but they can also create negative effects that impact the child's health and well-being.

Some of the common adverse effects of therapy for childhood leukaemia are:

1- Infection: Chemotherapy and other therapies may diminish the quantity of white blood cells, which help fight infections. This makes the youngster more prone to contracting infections from bacteria, viruses, or fungus. Infections may be severe and life-threatening, and may need hospitalisation and antibiotics. To prevent infections, the kid should avoid contact with others who are unwell, wash their hands regularly, and be vaccinated as suggested by their doctor.

2- Bleeding: Chemotherapy and other therapies may diminish the quantity of platelets, which help the blood clot. This makes the youngster more prone to bleed or bruise easily, particularly from the nose, gums, or skin. Bleeding may also occur inside, such as in the brain or stomach. Bleeding may be hazardous and may need transfusions of blood or platelets. To prevent bleeding, the kid should avoid activities that might cause harm, use a soft toothbrush and floss softly, and avoid aspirin and other medicines that can impair blood coagulation.

3- Anaemia: Chemotherapy and other therapies may diminish the quantity of red blood cells, which transport oxygen throughout the body. This creates anaemia, which is a condition when the blood does not have enough oxygen. Anaemia might make the youngster feel fatigued, weak, dizzy, or short of breath. Anaemia may also damage the heart and other organs. Anaemia may need infusions of red blood cells or medications that increase the creation of red blood cells. To deal with anaemia, the youngster should rest when required, consume a balanced diet, and drink lots of fluids.

4- Nausea and vomiting: Chemotherapy and other therapies may damage the stomach and intestines, producing nausea and vomiting. This might cause the youngster to lose their appetite, weight, and fluids. Nausea and vomiting might also influence the child's attitude and quality of life. Nausea and vomiting may be avoided or minimised by taking anti-nausea medicines before, during, or after therapy, as advised by the doctor. The youngster should also consume small, frequent, bland meals, avoid spicy, oily, or strong-smelling foods, and drink clear beverages like ginger ale.

5- Hair loss: Chemotherapy and other therapies may damage the hair follicles, causing the hair to fall out. This may affect the scalp, eyebrows, eyelashes, and other regions of the body. Hair loss may be unpleasant and impair the child's self-esteem and body image. Hair loss is normally transitory and the hair will come back following treatment, however it may be a different colour or texture. To deal with hair loss, the youngster may wear a hat, scarf, wig, or bandana, or shave their head if they desire. The youngster should also protect their scalp from the sun, cold, and illness, and use mild shampoo and conditioner.

6- Mouth sores: Chemotherapy and other therapies may destroy the cells that line the mouth, throat, and oesophagus, creating sores or ulcers. These may be painful and make it hard to eat, drink, or speak. Mouth sores may also raise the risk of infection and bleeding. Mouth sores may be avoided or cured by using mouthwashes or gels that include anaesthetic, antiseptic, or anti-inflammatory drugs, as recommended by the doctor. The youngster should also wash their teeth gently with a soft toothbrush, avoid alcohol, tobacco, and hot or acidic meals, and drink enough water.

7- Skin changes: Chemotherapy and other therapies might impact the skin, producing dryness, irritation, rash, or sensitivity to the sun. Some therapies, like radiation therapy or targeted therapy, may also cause redness, swelling, blistering, or peeling of the skin. Skin changes may be unpleasant and damage the child's look and self-confidence. Skin changes may be treated by using moisturisers, lotions, or ointments that include steroids, antibiotics, or antihistamines, as suggested by the doctor. The youngster should also avoid harsh soaps, fragrances, or cosmetics, wear loose-fitting garments made of cotton, and protect their skin from the sun, heat, and cold.

8- Growth and development: Chemotherapy and other therapies might impact the growth and development of the kid, particularly if they are administered at a young age or for a long period. Some therapies, such as radiation therapy or stem cell transplant, may potentially impair the fertility of the kid, which is their capacity to have children in the future. Growth and development may be tracked by measuring the height, weight, and bone age of the kid, and by evaluating their hormone levels and pubertal status. Growth and development may be encouraged by providing the kid growth hormone, thyroid hormone, or sex hormones, as required. Fertility may be maintained by freezing the sperm or eggs of the kid before treatment, if feasible.

These are some of the frequent adverse effects of therapy for childhood leukaemia, although there may be more, depending on the kind and amount of treatment, the age and health of the child, and the particular reaction of the kid. Not all children will suffer the same adverse effects, and certain side effects may be minor or severe, short-term or long-term. The doctor or nurse will discuss the probable adverse effects of each therapy, and how to avoid or treat them. The kid and their family should report any adverse effects or concerns to the doctor or nurse, and seek medical treatment if required. The kid and their family should also seek aid and support from the health care staff, other parents, or support groups, to deal with the physical and emotional obstacles of treatment.

Radiation treatment

Radiation therapy is a treatment that employs high-energy rays or particles to eliminate cancer cells. Radiation treatment is not generally required to cure leukaemia, however it may be utilised in some cases, such as:

- To prevent or cure the spread of leukaemia to the brain or testicles.

- To treat a tumour that is pushing on the windpipe.
- To prepare the body for a stem cell transplant.

Radiation treatment may be provided in many ways:

1- External radiation therapy: A machine focuses radiation beams at the location where the cancer cells are. This is done at a hospital or clinic, generally once a day for many days or weeks. The therapy itself is harmless, although some children may require anaesthesia to keep motionless.

2- Internal radiation therapy: A radioactive material is inserted within the body, near the cancer cells. This is done at a hospital, and the kid may need to remain there for a few days until the radiation is gone. This form of radiation treatment is seldom utilised for leukaemia.

3- Systemic radiation therapy: A radioactive material is administered by mouth or injection, and passes through the blood to reach the cancer cells. This is done at a hospital, and the kid may need to remain there for a few days until the radiation is gone. This sort of radiation treatment is occasionally used for leukaemia that has spread to the brain or spinal fluid.

Radiation treatment might have adverse effects that impact the child's health and well-being. The adverse effects depend on the dosage and location of the radiation, and may include:

- Hair loss in the treated area
- Skin abnormalities, such as redness, dryness, or peeling
- Nausea, vomiting, or diarrhoea
- Fatigue or weakness
- Infection or bleeding
- Mouth sores or difficulties swallowing
- Headache or eyesight issues
- Growth or development difficulties
- Fertility issues

The negative effects of radiation treatment are typically transitory and may be managed or avoided using drugs, creams, or other methods. The doctor or nurse will discuss the probable adverse effects of each therapy, and how to manage them. The kid and their family should report any adverse effects or concerns to the doctor or nurse, and seek medical treatment if required.

Radiation therapy may be an effective treatment for paediatric leukaemia, but it is not without dangers. Therefore, it is crucial to consider the advantages and dangers of each treatment choice, and discuss them with the child's medical team and family. The kid and their family should also seek aid and support from the health care staff, other parents, or support groups, to deal with the physical and emotional obstacles of treatment.

Stem cell transplantation

Stem cell transplantation (SCT) is a therapy option for certain children with leukaemia, a kind of blood cancer. Leukaemia arises when abnormal white blood cells grow out of control and push out the regular blood cells in the bone marrow. SCT tries to eliminate the leukaemia cells with heavy doses of chemotherapy and/or radiation treatment, and then replace the destroyed bone marrow with healthy stem cells from a donor.

Stem cells are immature cells that may grow into other kinds of blood cells, such as red blood cells, white blood cells, and platelets. They are present in the bone marrow, the blood, and the umbilical cord blood of newborn newborns. A donor for SCT might be a sibling, a relative, or an unrelated individual who has a matching tissue type (HLA type) with the patient. Sometimes, umbilical cord blood from a public bank may be utilised as well.

SCT is a difficult and hazardous treatment that needs specialist care and experience. It may produce major adverse effects, including infections, haemorrhage, graft-versus-host disease (GVHD), and organ damage.

Therefore, it is not suited for every kid with leukaemia. SCT is typically considered for children who have a high risk of recurrence, who do not react well to regular chemotherapy, or who suffer a second or later relapse. SCT may also be utilised for children with specific forms of leukaemia, such as Philadelphia chromosome-positive acute lymphoblastic leukaemia (ALL) or T-cell ALL.

The result of SCT relies on numerous aspects, such as the kind and stage of leukaemia, the source and quality of the stem cells, the conditioning regimen, the prevention and treatment of problems, and the patient's age and general health. SCT may give a possibility of cure for certain children with leukemia, but treatment also involves a risk of death and long-term consequences. Therefore, it is crucial to assess the advantages and hazards of SCT carefully, and to discuss them with the medical team and the family.

CHAPTER 4

Supporting the Child's Education and Development

Childhood leukaemia may influence the child's education and development in numerous ways. The youngster may miss school days, fall behind in their schoolwork, lose touch with their friends, or encounter learning challenges owing to sickness or treatment. The youngster may also suffer changes in their physical appearance, talents, or self-esteem. These problems may have a severe influence on the child's academic and social abilities, as well as their physical and emotional health.

However, there are strategies to assist the child to overcome these problems and promote their education and growth. Here are some recommendations on how to achieve that:

1- Help the kid remain connected to school: School is a vital aspect of the child's life, as it gives them a feeling of normality, regularity, and belonging. It also helps kids develop new skills, information, and values. Therefore, it is crucial to assist the child to remain connected to school as much as possible. This may be done by:

- Keeping in contact with the child's teachers and school workers. Inform them about the child's diagnosis, treatment, and requirements. Ask for their cooperation and support. Request for adjustments or changes in the child's curriculum, assignments, exams, or grades. Seek them advice on how to aid the youngster with their schooling.

- Encouraging the youngster to attend school whenever they are able to. Help them get ready for school by preparing their backpack, lunch, and medicine. Arrange for transportation or escort if required. Help them deal with any worry or fear they may have about going to school.

- Providing the child with other means of learning while they are unable to attend school. This may involve home tutoring, online classes, correspondence courses, or instructional resources. Help the youngster maintain a consistent schedule and routine for their learning. Monitor their development and give criticism and appreciation.

- Helping the children retain touch with their peers and friends. Encourage them to connect with them via phone conversations, video chats, emails, letters, or social media. Arrange for visits or playdates when feasible. Involve them in school events or activities, such as clubs, athletics, or festivals.

2- Attention the kid develops academic and social skills: The child may require additional attention and support to improve their academic and social abilities, particularly if they have missed a lot of school or have learning issues. This may be done by:

- Providing the child with extra learning materials or tools, such as books, workbooks, flashcards, games, or apps. Help them practise their reading, writing, maths, or other topics. Review their homework and tasks. Help them prepare for examinations or exams. Celebrate their triumphs and milestones.

- Encouraging the child to engage in extracurricular activities or interests, such as music, painting, theatre, or athletics. These may assist the child to express their creativity, abilities, and interests. They may also assist the child improve their physical, cognitive, and emotional abilities. They may also give the child an opportunity to mingle and make friends with people who share their hobbies.

- Teaching the kid social skills and etiquette, such as greeting, introducing, chatting, listening, sharing, collaborating, or resolving disagreements. Help children practise these skills in numerous circumstances and locations, such as at home, at school, or in public. Model these abilities yourself and give good encouragement and feedback. Help the youngster cope with any bullying, taunting, or prejudice they may experience because of their sickness or treatment.

- Helping the child to increase their self-confidence and self-esteem, such as by applauding their accomplishments, strengths, and traits. Help them develop reasonable and achievable objectives and encourage them to achieve them. Help them deal with any problems or setbacks they may experience. Help them understand and appreciate their individuality and importance. Help them accept and welcome any changes in their looks, talents, or lifestyle.

3- Help the kid maintain physical and mental health: The child's physical and mental health are crucial for their education and growth. Therefore, it is crucial to assist the child to maintain their physical and mental health as much as possible. This may be done by:

- Providing the kid with proper nourishment, water, rest, and cleanliness. Help them pursue a balanced and nutritious diet that matches their requirements and tastes. Help them drink enough water and fluids to keep hydrated. Help them get adequate sleep and rest to recuperate and replenish. Help them keep their body and surroundings clean and safe.

- Encouraging the child to exercise and be physically active, as long as it is safe and acceptable for them. Help them discover things that they love and can do, such as walking, bicycling, swimming, or dancing. Help them follow the advice and suggestions of their medical team about their physical activity. Monitor their symptoms and indications and seek medical assistance if required.

- Supporting the child's emotional and psychological well-being, such as by listening to their emotions and ideas. Help children express their feelings in healthy and productive ways, such as by talking, writing, painting, or playing. Help them manage with stress, anxiety, sadness, bereavement, trauma, or other challenges. Provide comfort, support, and reassurance. Seek professional assistance from a counsellor, therapist, psychologist, psychiatrist, or social worker if required.

4- Seek the role of teachers and schools: Teachers and schools play a significant role in assisting the child and the family throughout the child's sickness and treatment. They may offer the youngster with education, direction, and care. They may also give the family information, resources, and help. Therefore, it is necessary to examine the role of instructors and schools in assisting the kid and the family. This may be done by:

- Communicating with the instructors and school workers frequently and honestly. Share the child's diagnosis, treatment, and requirements. Ask for their cooperation and support. Request for adjustments or changes in the child's curriculum, assignments, exams, or grades. Seek them advice on how to aid the youngster with their schooling.
- Collaborating with the teachers and school personnel to produce an individualised education plan (IEP) or a 504 plan for the kid. These are legal papers that detail the child's educational objectives, services, and accommodations. They can assist the child to acquire the proper and required education and support they need and deserve.
- Appreciate the instructors and school personnel for their efforts and contributions. Thank them for their understanding and kindness. Provide them with comments and recommendations. Recognize and appreciate their efforts and triumphs. Maintain a pleasant and respectful connection with them.

Helping a sibling with childhood leukaemia

I know that having a brother or sister with cancer is very hard. You may feel many different emotions, like sadness, anger, fear, or guilt. These are all normal and okay. You are not alone in this.

Your sibling needs your love and support more than ever. You can help them in many ways, such as:

- Visiting them in the hospital or staying in touch through phone calls, texts, or video chats.
- Being patient and understanding when they are tired, sick, or in pain.
- Sharing your feelings and listening to theirs.
- Doing fun things together, like playing games, watching movies, or reading books.
- Helping them with school work or other activities.
- Encouraging them to stay positive and hopeful.

You are a very important part of your family. Your parents love you and care about you. They may be busy or stressed sometimes, but they are always there for you. You can talk to them about anything that is bothering you. They want to help you cope.

You can also find support from other people, like your friends, teachers, relatives, or counsellors. They can offer you comfort, advice, or a shoulder to cry on. You don't have to go through this alone.

Remember that you are a strong and brave person. You can overcome any challenge that comes your way. You and your sibling will get through this together.

Finding and Using Resources

Childhood leukaemia may bring numerous obstacles and hardships for the kid and the family. They may require different sorts of support and aid to deal with the sickness and treatment. Fortunately, there are numerous tools available that may aid them in many ways. These include:

1-Support groups: These are groups of individuals who share similar experiences or circumstances, such as having a kid with leukaemia or being a parent or caregiver of a child with leukaemia. They may give emotional support, practical guidance, knowledge, and encouragement to each other. They may also help minimise the emotions of isolation, loneliness, or stigma that the kid or the family may suffer. Support groups may be found online, via social media, websites, or forums, or offline, through hospitals, clinics, or community centres. Some examples of support groups are:

- *[Leukaemia & Lymphoma Society](https://www.lls.org/support/support-groups):* This is a nationwide organisation that provides online and in-person support groups for patients, families, and caregivers impacted by blood malignancies, such as leukaemia. They also give educational programs, financial help, and advocacy services.

[CancerCare](https://www.cancercare.org/support_groups): This is a nationwide organisation that provides online, telephone, and face-to-face support groups for individuals suffering with cancer, including children, teenagers, parents, and caregivers. They also give counselling, education, financial help, and recommendations.

- *[American Childhood Cancer Organization](https://www.acco.org/support-groups/):* This is a nationwide organisation that provides online and local support groups for families of children and adolescents with cancer. They also give information, resources, and advocacy.

2- Counselling services: These are professional services that may assist the kid and the family cope with the emotional, psychological, or social elements of living with leukaemia. They may give counselling, therapy, medicine, or other treatments to help them manage stress, anxiety, sadness, grief, trauma, or other concerns. They may also assist people enhance their communication, relationships, and coping abilities. Counselling services might be accessible via hospitals, clinics, schools, or community groups. Some examples of counselling services are:

- *[American Psychiatric Association](https://www.psychiatry.org/patients-families/find-a-psychiatrist):* This is a national organisation that can help people find a psychiatrist, who is a medical doctor who can diagnose and treat mental health conditions, such as depression, anxiety, or post-traumatic stress disorder. They may also prescribe medicine if required.

- *[American Psychological Association](https://www.apa.org/topics/find-help):* This is a national organisation that can help people find a psychologist, who is a licensed professional who can provide psychological testing, assessment, and treatment for mental health issues, such as stress, grief, or coping with illness. They may also give psychotherapy, which is a sort of talk therapy that can help individuals improve their attitudes, emotions, and actions.

- *[National Association of Social Workers](https://www.helpstartshere.org/find-a-social-worker/):* This is a national organisation that can help people find a social worker, who is a licensed professional who can provide counselling, case management, and referrals for social services, such as financial assistance, legal aid, or housing. They may also offer advocacy, education, and support for people, families, and communities.

3- Financial Help: This is a sort of assistance that may help the kid and the family pay for the medical and non-medical expenses of leukaemia treatment. These expenditures might include hospital bills, doctor fees, medicine, transportation, accommodation, food, or childcare. Financial aid may come from numerous sources, such as insurance, government programs, charities, foundations, or fundraisers. Some instances of financial aid are:

- *[Health Insurance](https://www.healthcare.gov/):* This is a form of insurance that may assist cover part or all of the medical expenditures linked to leukaemia treatment. Depending on the kind and amount of coverage, health insurance may pay for hospital stays, doctor visits, tests, operations, medicine, or equipment. Health insurance may be acquired via employers, commercial firms, or government programs, such as Medicaid or Medicare.

- *[Children's Health Insurance Program (CHIP)](https://www.insurekidsnow.gov/):* This is a federal and state program that offers low-cost or free health insurance for children and teenagers up to age 19, who do not qualify for Medicaid and whose families have poor or moderate income. CHIP may cover medical services, such as doctor visits, vaccines, medications, dental care, eye care, or mental health care.

- *[Patient Advocate Foundation](https://www.patientadvocate.org/):* This is a nationwide organisation that offers financial help, case management, and mediation services for people with chronic, life-threatening, or disabling illnesses, such as leukaemia. They may assist people obtain and afford health care, insurance, medicine, or other services. They may also assist patients address issues or appeals with insurance companies, employers, or creditors.

4- Legal guidance: This is a sort of advice that may assist the kid and the family understand and safeguard their rights and interests in regard to leukaemia treatment. These rights and interests might include health care access, insurance coverage, employment, education, handicap, or discrimination. Legal counsel may be acquired via attorneys, legal clinics, or advocacy organisations. Some instances of legal counsel are:

- [nationwide Cancer Legal assistance Network (NCLSN)](https://www.nclsn.org/): This is a nationwide network of organisations that offer free or low-cost legal assistance to persons afflicted by cancer, including children, parents, and caregivers. They may aid with concerns such as health care access, insurance, employment, education, housing, or estate preparation.

- [Cancer and Careers](https://www.cancerandcareers.org/en): This is a nationwide organisation that offers information, resources, and support for working individuals with cancer, including parents and caregivers. They may aid with concerns such as disclosure, privacy, discrimination, leave, or accommodations at work.

- [The 504 Plan](https://www.understood.org/en/school-learning/special-services/504-plan/the-difference-between-ieps-and-504-plans): This is a legal document that details the accommodations and assistance that a child with a condition, such as leukaemia, may require to succeed in school. These accommodations and services might include more time, modified assignments, tutoring, counselling, or transportation. The 504 plan is distinct from the individualised education plan (IEP), which is for children who require special education.

5- Educational resources: These are items that may give knowledge, education, and awareness regarding leukaemia and its treatment. These resources may include books, brochures, websites, films, podcasts, or webinars. They may assist the kid and the family to understand more about the condition, the treatment choices, the side effects, the complications, and the long-term impacts. They may also help patients manage with the emotional, social, and practical elements of life with leukaemia. Some examples of instructional resources are:

- *[National Cancer Institute (NCI)](https://www.cancer.gov/types/leukemia):* This is a government institution that conducts and supports research, training, and teaching on cancer, including leukaemia. They give complete and authoritative information about leukaemia, such as its causes, symptoms, diagnosis, treatment, prevention, and statistics. They also provide papers, films, podcasts, and webinars on many issues linked to leukaemia and cancer.

- *[American Cancer Society (ACS)](https://www.cancer.org/cancer/leukemia-in-children.html):* This is a national organisation that finances and conducts research, education, and advocacy on cancer, including leukaemia. They give extensive and current information about leukaemia in children, such as its kinds, stages, risk factors, testing, therapies, survival rates, and follow-up care. They also provide support services, activities, and events for children and families impacted by leukaemia and cancer.

-

[KidsHealth](https://kidshealth.org/en/parents/leukemia.html): This is a website that gives information, advice, and guidance on health, behaviour, and development for children, teenagers, and parents. They include easy-to-understand and age-appropriate information about leukaemia, such as what it is, how it is treated, how it affects the body, and how to deal with it. They also provide interactive elements, such as games, quizzes, films, and tales.

To get access to these resources, the kid and the family may do the following:

1- Ask for suggestions and referrals from their medical team, social worker, counsellor, or other health care experts. They may have expertise or knowledge of the best and most relevant resources for the kid and the family's needs and preferences.

2-Search online or offline for the materials that interest them. They may use keywords, filters, ratings, reviews, or testimonies to narrow down their search and select the most relevant and credible resources. They may also compare and contrast various resources and evaluate which ones give the greatest benefits and advantages for them.

3- Contact or visit the resources that they have chosen. They may ask questions, seek information, or make appointments with the resources. They may also verify the credentials, qualifications, and reputation of the resources. They may also evaluate whether the materials are accessible, inexpensive, and available for them.

4-Try out the materials and see how they work for them. They may monitor and assess the results, effects, and satisfaction of utilising the resources. They may also submit comments, recommendations, or concerns to the resources. They may also swap or cease utilising the resources if they are not happy or comfortable with them.

CHAPTER 5

Long-Term Outlook and Follow-Up Care

Childhood leukaemia is a severe and life-threatening illness, yet it is also one of the most treatable and curable kinds of cancer. With breakthroughs in diagnosis, therapy, and supportive care, the survival rates and quality of life for children with leukaemia have improved dramatically over the years. However, there are still certain obstacles and hazards that the kid and the family may encounter once the therapy is done. These include the chance of recurrence, late effects, and ambiguity. Therefore, it is necessary to have frequent and long-term follow-up treatment and to plan for the future and live with uncertainty. Here are some points to consider:

1- Survival rates: Survival rates are statistics that reflect how probable a person is to live a specific amount of time after being diagnosed with an illness, such as leukaemia. They are based on the results of huge groups of persons who had the same kind and stage of leukaemia in the past. They are not perfect forecasts of what will happen to a given kid, since they do not take into account the individual characteristics, such as age, health, reaction to therapy, or genetic abnormalities. However, they may offer a basic notion of the prognosis and outlook for a kid with leukaemia. According to the American Cancer Society, the 5-year survival rate for children with acute lymphoblastic leukaemia (ALL), the most prevalent kind of leukaemia in children, is around 90%. The 5-year survival rate for children with acute myeloid leukaemia (AML), the second most frequent kind of leukaemia in children, is around 65%. The 5-year survival rate for children with chronic myeloid leukaemia (CML), an uncommon kind of leukaemia in children, is around 85%. The 5-year survival rate for children with chronic lymphocytic leukaemia (CLL), another rare kind of leukaemia in children, is not known, since it is exceedingly uncommon in children and mainly affects older individuals.

2- Recurrence: Recurrence is the recurrence of leukaemia after it has been treated and gone into remission. Remission is the absence of signs or symptoms of leukaemia, or the decrease of leukaemia cells to a very low level. Recurrence may happen at any moment, although it is more likely to happen during the first few years following therapy. The probability of recurrence relies on numerous variables, such as the type and subtype of leukaemia, the first response to therapy, the existence of specific genetic abnormalities, or the emergence of complications or infections.

Recurrence may be recognized by frequent testing and examinations, such as blood tests, bone marrow tests, or imaging tests. If recurrence is suspected or confirmed, the child may need to receive additional treatment, such as chemotherapy, targeted therapy, immunotherapy, or stem cell transplant. The treatment choices and results for recurrence depend on the kind and degree of recurrence, the prior therapy, and the child's general health and condition.

3- Late effects: Late effects are health concerns that may arise months or years after the treatment for leukemia is done. They are caused by the harm or alterations that the leukemia or its treatment may have caused to the body's organs, tissues, or functions. They may influence the physical, mental, or emotional wellbeing of the kid. Some examples of late consequences are:
- Growth and development issues, such as delayed puberty, small height, or learning challenges.
- Fertility difficulties, such as low sperm count, ovarian failure, or early menopause.
- Heart disorders, such as cardiomyopathy, arrhythmia, or coronary artery disease.
- Lung disorders, such as pulmonary fibrosis, bronchiolitis obliterans, or asthma.
- Bone issues, such as osteoporosis, osteonecrosis, or fractures.
- Kidney issues, such as renal failure, hypertension, or proteinuria.

- Thyroid issues, such as hypothyroidism, hyperthyroidism, or thyroid cancer.
- Eye disorders, such as cataracts, glaucoma, or dry eyes.
- Hearing difficulties, such as hearing loss, tinnitus, or ear infections.
- Dental disorders, such as tooth decay, gum disease, or oral cancer.
- Skin concerns, such as skin cancer, scarring, or radiation dermatitis.
- Nervous system disorders, such as stroke, convulsions, or peripheral neuropathy.
- Immune system disorders, such as infections, autoimmune illnesses, or graft-versus-host disease.
- Psychological difficulties, such as anxiety, depression, post-traumatic stress disorder, or survivor guilt.
- Second malignancies, such as leukemia, lymphoma, or solid tumors.

4- Quality of life: Quality of life is a measure of how well a person is able to function and enjoy their life, despite having a sickness or its treatment. It may be impacted by various things, such as the physical, mental, emotional, social, and spiritual components of the person's health and well-being. Quality of life may vary from person to person, and from period to time, based on the individual's requirements, tastes, values, and aspirations. Quality of life may be increased by numerous tactics, such as:

- Maintaining a healthy lifestyle, such as eating healthily, exercising, sleeping, and resting.
- Seeking medical treatment and follow-up, such as taking medicine, following instructions, and attending appointments.
- Managing symptoms and side effects, such as pain, nausea, exhaustion, or anxiety.
- Seeking support and help, such as from family, friends, professionals, or organisations.
-    - Pursuing interests and activities, such as hobbies, education, job, or volunteering.
- Expressing emotions and ideas, such as via talking, writing, painting, or playing.
- Finding meaning and purpose, such as by creating objectives, making plans, or assisting others.

5- Follow-up care: Follow-up care is the continuous and regular care that the kid and the family get after the treatment for leukaemia is done. It is crucial to have follow-up care to monitor the child's health and well-being, to identify and treat any recurrence or late consequences, and to enhance the child's quality of life. Follow-up care might include:

- Physical examinations, such as evaluating the child's height, weight, blood pressure, pulse, and temperature.

- Blood tests, such as testing the child's blood cell counts, liver and kidney function, hormone levels, and immune system activity.
- Bone marrow testing, such as evaluating the child's bone marrow cells for any symptoms of leukaemia or other abnormalities.
- Imaging testing, such as evaluating the child's chest, abdomen, or brain for any tumours or infections.
- Other tests, such as assessing the child's heart, lung, or hearing function, or screening for any second malignancies.
- Vaccinations, such as providing the youngster the appropriate immunizations to avoid infections and illnesses.
- Medications, such as providing the kid the necessary medications to prevent or treat any problems or infections.
- Referrals, such as sending the kid to other experts or services for additional examination or treatment.
- Education, such as giving the kid and the family with information and guidance on how to deal with leukaemia and its treatment, and how to avoid or manage any recurrence or late consequences.
- Support, such as supplying the kid and the family emotional, psychological, social, or spiritual support and direction.

6- Preparing for the future and living with uncertainty: The future might be unknown and unexpected for the kid and the family when the treatment for leukaemia is ended. They may have numerous questions, worries, or anxieties about what will happen next, such as if the leukaemia will come back, whether the kid will have any late consequences, or whether the child will be able to live a normal and happy life. These sensations are acceptable and reasonable, but they may also induce tension, worry, or despair. Therefore, it is vital to plan for the future and manage uncertainty in a healthy and good manner. Some ways to do that are:

- Planning forward, such as developing a long-term follow-up plan with the medical team, maintaining a record of the child's medical history and treatment, and updating the child's legal and financial papers, such as wills, insurance, or guardianship.
- Living in the now, such as concentrating on the child's current health and well-being, appreciating the child's successes and milestones, and celebrating the child's survival and recovery.
- Hoping for the best, such as being positive and confident in the child's prognosis and outlook, trusting the child's medical team and treatment, and believing in the child's strength and perseverance.

- Preparing for the worst, such as being realistic and aware of the probable dangers and obstacles, having a backup plan and a support structure, and requesting aid and support when required.
- Finding balance, such as accepting the uncertainty and the lack of control, but also taking action and making choices, being flexible and adaptable, but also being consistent and stable, and being cautious and careful, but also being adventurous and curious.

Nutrition

Nutrition is a crucial element of healing for children with leukaemia who have had treatment. Treatment might alter the child's appetite, digestion, metabolism, and immune system, which can lead to nutritional difficulties such as weight loss, malnutrition, infections, and poor development. Therefore, it is crucial to offer appropriate and balanced nourishment to assist the child's recovery and growth.

According to the Leukaemia and Lymphoma Society (LLS), a nutritious diet for children with leukaemia should include:

- A mix of fruits and vegetables, which should make up roughly 50% of most meals
- Whole grains, such as oatmeal, brown rice, quinoa, and whole wheat bread
- Fat-free or low-fat dairy products, such as milk, yoghourt, and cheese
- Low-fat protein sources, such as chicken, fish, eggs, beans, almonds, and soy - Healthy oils, such as olive, canola, or sunflower oil

Some children may develop unique nutritional adverse effects from therapy, such as nausea, vomiting, constipation, diarrhoea, mouth sores, taste changes, weight gain, or weight loss. In these circumstances, the child's diet may need to be changed to fit their specific requirements and preferences. Some common recommendations to manage these negative effects are:

- For nausea and vomiting, eat small, frequent meals; avoid spicy, oily, or strong-smelling foods; drink clear beverages or chew on ice chips; and take anti-nausea drugs as recommended.

- For constipation, drink lots of fluids; consume high-fibre meals, such as fruits, vegetables, and whole grains; and take laxatives or stool softeners as advised.

- For diarrhoea, drink lots of fluids to prevent dehydration; consume bland, low-fibre meals, such as white rice, bananas, applesauce, and toast; and avoid dairy products, caffeine, alcohol, and sweets.

- For mouth sores, consume soft, moist meals, such as soups, smoothies, mashed potatoes, and scrambled eggs; avoid acidic, spicy, salty, or crunchy foods; and rinse the mouth with salt water or baking soda solution.

- For taste changes, try different spices, sauces, or marinades to enhance the flavour of meals; use plastic utensils or glasses to reduce metallic taste; and avoid products that taste terrible or cause discomfort.

- For weight gain, restrict consumption of high-calorie, high-fat, and high-sugar foods, such as fast food, fried food, sweets, and soda; pick low-calorie, nutrient-dense foods, such as fruits, vegetables, lean protein, and whole grains; and increase physical activity as tolerated.

- For weight reduction, increase consumption of high-calorie, high-protein foods, such as cheese, almonds, peanut butter, eggs, milk, and yoghourt; add additional calories and protein to foods, such as butter, cream, cheese, honey, jam, or powdered milk; and eat often and snack between meals.

It is crucial to contact a certified dietitian or a nutritionist who can give tailored counsel and assistance for the child's dietary requirements. They may also monitor the child's growth and development, and offer supplements or special formulations if required. A well-balanced diet may help the kid deal with therapy, reduce problems, and improve recovery.

Conclusion

Coping with Childhood Leukaemia: A Practical and Supportive Handbook for Families, Friends and Teachers is a comprehensive guide for anyone who is affected by a child's diagnosis of leukaemia or lymphoma. The book gives clear and accurate medical information, as well as practical guidance on how to cope with the emotional, social, and financial obstacles of cancer treatment and surviving. The book also offers experiences from families who have gone through the journey of children with leukaemia or lymphoma, bringing hope and inspiration to readers. The book is a helpful resource for parents, siblings, relatives, friends, teachers, and healthcare professionals who wish to understand and assist a kid with cancer.